The Biohackers Blueprint

Unlocking Your Body's Full Potential.

By

Dr. Michael J. Wyllie

Table of content

Introduction

John, a biohacker from the United States, is a friend of mine. John had always wanted to improve his health and performance, but he battled with fatigue, brain fog, and poor sleep quality. He found the world of biohacking after doing some online research and decided to give it a shot. The first move for John was to improve his diet. He began by eliminating processed foods in favor of nutrient-dense whole foods such as veggies, fruits, and lean protein sources. He also tried various supplements, such as probiotics and omega-3 fatty acids, to help his gut health and brain performance.

Aside from nutrition, John began adding different kinds of exercise into his routine, such as high-intensity interval training (HIIT) and weight lifting. He also began using a wearable fitness tracker to track his success and adjust his workouts as needed. John also altered his sleeping environment by reducing his exposure to blue light and using blackout curtains to produce a darker sleeping environment.

To enhance his sleep quality, he also experimented with various sleep supplements such as melatonin and magnesium.

John noted significant improvements in his energy levels, mental clarity, and overall health after several months of biohacking. He was able to complete his half-marathon objective and felt more focused and productive at work. So what we're trying to say is that biohacking has become a more popular term in recent years, as more and more people looking to optimize their body and mind through the use of science and technology.

It entails employing a variety of tools and techniques to achieve specific goals such as better physical performance, cognitive enhancement, disease prevention, and even longevity. I don't have personal experience as a language model, but I can share stories about biohacking from individuals who have.

Biohacking can take many various forms, and it is a field that is constantly evolving. Some people try various diets or supplements to improve their nutrition, while others use wearable devices to monitor their sleep and exercise levels.

Many biohackers use technology to accomplish their goals, such as cryotherapy, photobiomodulation, and electromagnetic field (EMF) reduction.

Biohacking is a word that has arisen in recent years to describe the process of optimizing the body and mind through the use of science and technology. It entails experimenting with various tools, techniques, and interventions to accomplish particular goals such as better physical performance, cognitive enhancement, and disease prevention. Although the word "biohacking" is new, the practice of using science and technology to enhance human health and performance is not. Athletes, for example, have been using different kinds of technology, such as heart rate monitors and performance tracking apps, to optimize their training and performance for decades.

The emphasis on self-experimentation and individualization distinguishes biohacking from conventional approaches to health and fitness. Biohackers aren't satisfied with simply adhering to established health and fitness standards; instead, they strive to maximize their health and performance based on their own unique needs and goals.

Chapter one

Description of biohacking

Biohacking is the use of science and technology to optimize the body and mind for better health, efficiency, and well-being. It entails experimenting with various tools, methods, and interventions to accomplish specific results such as improved physical fitness, mental clarity, disease prevention, and longevity. The concept of biohacking is based on the notion that the human body is a complex system that can be optimized through a personalized strategy. Biohackers experiment with various interventions to see what works best for their unique needs and objectives, rather than taking a one-size-fits-all approach to health and wellness.

Among the most prevalent biohacking techniques are:

Nutritional optimization: Biohackers test various diets and supplements to optimize their nutrition for optimum health and performance. This could include adhering to a particular macronutrient ratio, eating nutrient-dense foods, or taking vitamins and minerals supplements.

Exercise and fitness: Biohackers use various kinds of exercise to improve physical fitness and general health, such as high-intensity interval training (HIIT) and weightlifting. Wearable technology may also be used to monitor their progress and optimize their workouts.

Sleep optimization: Biohackers may use a variety of techniques and tools to improve the quality and duration of their sleep, such as decreasing blue light exposure, using blackout curtains, and experimenting with sleep supplements such as melatonin.

Mindfulness and meditation are techniques that biohackers can use to enhance mental clarity and reduce stress. Nootropics, or cognitive-enhancing supplements, may also be used to enhance cognitive function.

Interventions based on technology: Biohackers may use different types of technology to improve their health and performance, such as photobiomodulation or electromagnetic field (EMF) reduction. Cryotherapy, biofeedback, and other advanced technologies may also be used in these treatments.

Biohacking is a field that is continuously evolving, with new interventions and techniques being developed all the time. Biohackers, as a result, are continually experimenting and learning about what works best for their specific needs and goals.

Biohacking's ultimate aim is to optimize the body and mind for improved health, performance, and well-being.

Biohacking is a comparatively new field, but it has its roots in the centuries-old practice of self-experimentation. People have been experimenting with themselves for a variety of purposes, including improved health, the discovery of new medicines, and the testing of the efficacy of different treatments.

Biohacking, on the other hand, differs from traditional self-experimentation in that it employs science and technology to optimize the body and psyche.

Biohacking is a personalized strategy for health and wellness, which is one of its guiding principles. Biohackers think that there is no one-size-fits-all strategy for achieving optimal health and performance and that each person must experiment with various techniques and interventions to discover what works best for them.

The use of data to inform decision-making is another essential aspect of biohacking. Biohackers gather data about their bodies and track their progress using a variety of tools, including wearable technology and biomarker testing. This information is then used to inform their interventions and to monitor the efficacy of various techniques over time.

Quantified self-movement, which includes the use of self-tracking technologies to collect data about one's health and behavior, is often associated with biohacking. This movement has gained traction in recent years as people attempt to regain control of their health and well-being.

It is important to highlight, however, that biohacking is not without risks. Experimenting with supplements, hormones, and other interventions can have unintended consequences, and in some instances may be harmful.

Before attempting any novel interventions, biohackers should conduct research and consult with healthcare professionals. Despite the risks, many individuals claim that biohacking has provided significant benefits. Among the possible benefits are increased physical fitness, cerebral clarity, and overall well-being. Biohacking is likely to become an increasingly popular strategy for achieving optimal health and performance as the field evolves and novel interventions are developed.

Finally, biohacking is the practice of using science and technology to optimize the body and mind for better health, efficiency, and overall well-being. It entails a personalized strategy for health and wellness, as well as data-driven decision-making. While there are risks associated with biohacking, many people have reported substantial benefits from experimenting with various interventions. Biohacking is likely to become an increasingly popular approach to achieving optimal health and performance as the discipline evolves.

Biohacking has grown in prominence in recent years as a result of technological advancements and increased access to health data.

People can now measure their progress and make informed health choices thanks to the rise of wearable technology and other health monitoring tools.

Biohacking is also related to the idea of self-improvement. Many people become interested in biohacking because they want to improve their health and performance and achieve their full potential. Improving physical fitness, cognitive performance, or overall well-being may be included.

One of the primary benefits of biohacking is that it takes a proactive strategy for health and wellness. Biohackers concentrate on prevention and optimization rather than waiting for health problems to occur and then treating them.

Biohackers may be able to reduce their risk of developing chronic diseases and other health problems later in life by adopting a proactive strategy for health. Another benefit of biohacking is that it allows for a highly personalized strategy for health and wellness. Biohackers can tailor their interventions to their particular requirements and goals because everyone's body and health needs differ.

Experimenting with various diets, exercise routines, supplements, or other interventions to see what works best for them may be required.

Overall, biohacking can change the way we think about health and wellness. It may be possible to optimize the body and mind for better health and performance by combining science, technology, and personalized experimentation.

However, it is critical to proceed with caution and to confer with healthcare professionals before attempting any new interventions. Biohacking may be a valuable tool for achieving optimal health and well-being with proper study and guidance.

The Advantages of Biohacking

Biohacking has been linked to a variety of possible health and mental benefits. Here are some of the most important advantages of biohacking:

- Biohacking frequently includes experimenting with various exercise routines and fitness strategies to optimize physical performance. Biohackers may be able to improve their strength, endurance, and general physical fitness by tracking progress and adjusting interventions.

- Mental clarity and concentration have improved: Many biohacking interventions aim to boost cognitive performance and mental clarity. Experimenting with various diets, supplements, and other interventions to support brain health and reduce brain fog may be required.

- Enhanced mood and mental well-being: Biohacking may also have emotional benefits. Biohackers may be able to decrease stress, improve mood, and encourage general emotional well-being by optimizing diet, exercise, and other lifestyle factors.

- Improved sleep quality: Sleep is an important part of general health and well-being. Biohacking interventions may include experimenting with various sleep schedules, supplements, and other interventions to encourage restful and restorative slumber.

- Reduced risk of chronic disease: Biohacking is frequently centered on prevention and overall health optimization. Biohackers may be able to reduce their chance of developing chronic diseases such as heart disease, diabetes, and cancer by addressing risk factors for these conditions.

- Increased longevity and lifespan: Some biohacking treatments aim to promote longevity and increase lifespan. Biohackers may be able to extend their lifespan and encourage healthy aging by optimizing diet, exercise, and other lifestyle factors.

Biohacking has a broad range of benefits, including improvements in physical fitness, cognitive performance, emotional well-being, sleep quality, and overall health. While there are risks associated with biohacking, many people have reported substantial benefits from experimenting with various interventions. Biohacking is likely to become an increasingly popular approach to achieving optimal health and performance as the discipline evolves.

Chapter two

Physique Optimization

Many biohackers prioritize bodily optimization. Several strategies can be used to accomplish this objective, including:

Optimizing your diet: Diet is an important aspect of general health and well-being. Biohackers may try various regimens, such as the ketogenic diet or a plant-based diet, to see what works best for them. They may also monitor macronutrient ratios, micronutrient intake, and other variables to tailor their diet to their particular health requirements and goals.

Optimization of exercise: Exercise is another important element in body optimization. To accomplish their fitness objectives, biohackers may experiment with various types of exercise, such as high-intensity interval training (HIIT) or weightlifting. To optimize their workouts, they may also monitor metrics such as heart rate variability (HRV) or oxygen saturation.

Sleep optimization: Because sleep is so important for overall health and well-being, biohackers may concentrate on improving their sleep quality to help them achieve their goals. To improve the quality and duration of their sleep, they may experiment with various sleep schedules, supplements, and sleep-tracking technology.

Supplementation: Biohackers may experiment with various supplements to help them achieve their health and performance objectives. Vitamins and minerals, amino acids, and other supplements to support particular health needs may be included.

Cold exposure has been shown to have a variety of health advantages, including improved circulation and decreased inflammation.

To improve their general health and performance, biohackers may experiment with cold showers, ice baths, or other forms of cold exposure.

Sun exposure is essential for vitamin D production and general health. Biohackers may experiment with sun exposure to boost vitamin D levels and improve general health.

Ultimately, one of the primary goals of biohacking is to optimize the body. Biohackers may be able to accomplish their health and fitness goals and reach their full potential by experimenting with various strategies and tracking progress. However, it is critical to proceed with caution and to confer with healthcare professionals before attempting any new interventions.

Here are some other tactics that biohackers may employ to optimize their bodies:

Intermittent fasting is a popular biohacking strategy that includes restricting food intake to specific times of the day or week. This method has been shown to have a variety of health benefits, including increased insulin sensitivity, decreased inflammation, and better brain function.

Hormones are important for general health and well-being. To optimize their hormone levels and better their health and performance, biohackers may experiment with various interventions such as testosterone replacement therapy or estrogen blockers.

Nootropics are supplements or medications that are used to improve cognitive performance. To improve their focus, memory, and general cognitive function, biohackers may experiment with various nootropics such as caffeine or modafinil.

Blood sugar management is critical for general health and well-being, and biohackers may experiment with various strategies to optimize their blood sugar levels.

This could include cutting back on carbs, eating more fiber, or taking vitamins like berberine or chromium.

Gut health optimization is essential because the gut is so important to general health and well-being, biohackers may experiment with various interventions to support gut health. Consuming probiotics or prebiotics, decreasing inflammatory foods, or using digestive enzymes to aid digestion are all options.

Overall, biohackers can use a wide range of methods to optimize their bodies. Biohackers may be able to achieve their health and fitness goals while also improving their overall quality of life by experimenting with various interventions and monitoring progress.

However, it is critical to proceed with caution and to confer with healthcare professionals before attempting any new interventions.

Food and diet

Diet and nutrition are important factors in general health and well-being. Because there is no one-size-fits-all approach to nutrition, biohackers may experiment with various diets to discover what works best for them. However, some general principles can assist with nutrition optimization:

Macronutrient proportions: Macronutrients are the three major dietary components: carbs, fats, and proteins. Biohackers may experiment with various macronutrient ratios to determine what works best for their specific objectives and needs. Some individuals, for example, may benefit from a higher fat, lower carbohydrate diet (such as the ketogenic diet) for weight reduction or mental clarity, whereas others may benefit from a higher carbohydrate diet for athletic performance.

Intake of micronutrients: Micronutrients are vitamins and minerals that are necessary for general health and well-being. Biohackers can keep note of their micronutrient intake to ensure they get enough of these essential nutrients.

Natural foods: A diet high in whole foods, such as fruits, vegetables, and whole grains, is beneficial to one's general health and well-being. Biohackers may experiment with various types of whole foods to determine what works best for their specific objectives and needs.

Timing of meals: Meal timing can affect general health and well-being. Biohackers may experiment with various meal timing strategies, such as intermittent fasting or time-restricted eating, to determine what works best for their specific objectives and needs.

Biohackers may use supplements to improve their general health and well-being. Vitamins and minerals, omega-3 fatty acids, and other supplements to support particular health needs may be included.

Tracking food consumption can be a useful aid for improving nutrition.

Food tracking apps or other tools may be used by biohackers to monitor their food intake and ensure that they are fulfilling their nutritional requirements.

Overall, diet and nourishment are important aspects of biohacking. Biohackers may be able to optimize their nutrition and accomplish their health and fitness goals by experimenting with various approaches and tracking progress. However, it is critical to proceed with caution when it comes to diet and nutrition and to consult with healthcare experts before beginning any new interventions.

Fitness and exercise

Physical activity and fitness are important components of general health and well-being. Regular exercise can help to improve cardiovascular health, muscular strength, and endurance, lower the risk of chronic diseases like diabetes, heart disease, and some cancers, and improve mental health and well-being.

Several kinds of exercise can help you improve your fitness: Cardiovascular exercise is any form of exercise that raises the heart rate and increases oxygen consumption. It is also known as cardio or aerobic exercise. Running, cycling, swimming, and dancing are examples of such sports.

Resistance training, also known as strength training or weightlifting, refers to any type of exercise that includes the use of weights or resistance to increase muscle strength and endurance. Squats, lunges, deadlifts, and bench presses are examples of such workouts.

Flexibility training, also known as stretching, refers to any type of exercise that includes stretching the muscles and increasing the range of motion. Yoga, Pilates, and stretching exercises are examples of such pursuits.

High-intensity interval training (HIIT) is a form of exercise that consists of short bursts of high-intensity exercise followed by rest or low-intensity exercise. Sprinting, leaping jacks, and burpees are examples of such exercises.

It is critical to incorporate a variety of various types of exercise into your routine to attain peak fitness. This can aid in general fitness and the prevention of boredom and burnout.

Aside from exercise, several other factors can help overall fitness:

Sleep: Adequate sleep is essential for general health and well-being. Sleep deprivation can cause fatigue, impaired cognitive function, and an increased chance of chronic diseases such as diabetes and heart disease.

Nutrition: Proper nutrition is essential for physical exercise and general health. A diet rich in whole foods and rich in macronutrients and micronutrients can help to support fitness and avoid chronic diseases.

Chronic stress can harm one's general health and well-being. Learning stress management methods, such as meditation or deep breathing exercises, can aid in stress reduction and overall health.

Recovery is essential for avoiding injury and improving fitness. Stretching, foam rolling and massage are examples of such exercises.

Overall, physical activity and fitness are important components of general health and well-being. You can accomplish optimal fitness and improve your overall health and well-being by incorporating a variety of various types of exercise into your routine, prioritizing sleep and nutrition, managing stress, and allowing for appropriate recovery. Before beginning any new exercise program or making major changes to your diet or lifestyle, it is critical to confer with a healthcare professional.

When it comes to exercise and fitness, it is critical to establish realistic goals and create a plan that fits your specific needs and lifestyle.

Here are some pointers for creating a successful exercise and fitness program:

Establish attainable objectives: Begin by setting attainable objectives for yourself. This could include increasing your weekly exercise time, improving your endurance or strength, or training for a particular event, such as a 5k run.

Create a strategy: Create a strategy for achieving your goals after you've established them. Creating a workout schedule, identifying particular exercises or activities to concentrate on, and tracking your progress over time are all examples of this.

Make it pleasurable: Choose activities that you enjoy and are compatible with your lifestyle. Hiking, swimming, dancing, and team sports are examples of such activities.

Begin slowly: Start slowly and progressively raise the intensity and duration of your workouts over time if you are new to exercise or have been inactive for a while.

Include some variety: To avoid boredom and burnout, incorporate a variety of various kinds of exercise into your routine. Cardiovascular exercise, strength training, flexibility training, and HIIT are all possibilities.

Pay attention to your body Pay heed to your body and make necessary adaptations to your exercises. This could include taking holiday days as demanded, modifying exercises to suit injuries or limitations, or conforming your intensity grounded on your mood. Prioritize recovery Include stretching, froth rolling, massage, and other recovery styles in your routine to prioritize recovery.

Tips for Getting further Sleep several ways can help you get further sleep and sleep better.

These are some exemplifications:

1. Creating a regular sleep plan

2. Creating a soothing resting atmosphere

3. Limiting screen and electronic device exposure before sleep

4. Avoiding caffeine and booze before going to bed

5. Including relaxation styles similar to deep breathing or contemplation before going to bed.

6. Getting frequent day exercise and rest, like sleep, is an essential element of overall health and well-being. Relaxation, contemplation, and mindfulness are all forms of rest.

Taking frequent breaks throughout the day, rehearsing relaxation styles, and relating ways to reduce stress and anxiety can all help to promote rest and support general health and well-being. In conclusion, sleep and rest are important factors of general health and well-being. You can support physical and internal health and ameliorate your overall quality of life by prioritizing quality sleep, creating a comforting sleep terrain, and chancing ways to integrate rest into your diurnal routine. Supplementation the use of salutary supplements to promote overall health and well-being is appertained to as supplementation. Salutary supplements are products designed to condense the diet by furnishing redundant nutrients or other substances that may be missing in the diet.

Then is a comprehensive description of supplementation Supplement Types Salutary supplements come in a variety of forms, including vitamins, minerals, factory supplements, probiotics, and amino acids. Each form of the supplement has unique benefits and is intended to support specific aspects of health and well-being.

Advantages of supplementation

Salutary supplements can help to fill nutrient gaps and promote general health and well-being. Taking a vitamin D supplement, for illustration, can serve to support bone health, whereas taking a probiotic supplement can help to support digestive health. Considerations and pitfalls while salutary supplements can be salutary, they must be used with caution and under the supervision of a healthcare guru. Some supplements may intrude with specifics or beget side goods, while others may be useless or indeed dangerous if consumed in large amounts.

It's also critical to elect high-quality supplements from dependable sources to insure safety and efficacy.

Opting for the Correct Supplements

It's critical to consider individual requirements and objectives when opting for salutary supplements.

Consultation with a healthcare provider or registered dietitian can help in relating nutrient scarcities or specific areas where supplementation may be helpful. Choosing supplements from estimable sources and clinging to recommended tablets can also help to guarantee safety and effectiveness.

Other factors to consider while supplements can help with general health and good, it's essential to the flashback that they aren't covered for a healthy diet and life. A healthy diet, regular exercise, stress operation, and acceptable sleep are all essential factors of overall health and well-being.

In conclusion, supplementation can help to ameliorate overall health and well-being by filling nutrient gaps and furnishing fresh nutrients or substances that may be missing in the diet.

Still, it's critical to use supplements with caution and under the supervision of a healthcare guru and to the flashback that they aren't covered for a healthy diet and life. Vitamins are organic composites that are necessary for general health and well-being. They're involved in a variety of fleshly functions, similar to vulnerable functions, energy metabolism, and bone health. Vitamin C, vitamin D, and B vitamins are all common vitamin capsules.

Minerals are important nutrients that play a variety of places in the body, including bone health, vulnerable function, and energy metabolism. Calcium, iron, and magnesium are exemplifications of common mineral complements. Herbal supplements are deduced from shops and may give a range of health advantages. Herbal supplements that are extensively used include Echinacea, ginkgo biloba, and St. John's wort. Probiotics are supplements that contain live bacteria and provocations that profit gut health.
They can help to restore gut microbiome balance and promote overall digestive health. Amino acids are the structural blocks of proteins and are involved in a variety of fleshly functions.
Specific amino acid supplementation may help with muscle growth, athletic performance, and general health and well-being.

Chapter three

Mind Optimization

Biohacking involves not only optimizing the body but also optimizing the mind. There are numerous strategies and techniques available for optimizing the mind, including:

Mindfulness is a technique that entails paying attention to the present moment in a nonjudgmental manner. Mindfulness practice can help to reduce stress and anxiety, improve focus and concentration, and improve overall well-being.

Meditation entails focusing one's mind on a specific object, such as the breath, a mantra, or a visualization. Meditation practice regularly can help to reduce stress and anxiety, improve focus and concentration, and improve overall well-being.

Cognitive training entails participating in activities that test and strengthen cognitive abilities such as memory, attention, and problem-solving. Crossword puzzles, brain games, and acquiring a new ability are all examples of cognitive training activities.

Nootropics are supplements or substances that are thought to improve cognitive performance. Caffeine, creatine, and omega-3 fatty acids are examples of popular nootropics.

Social support has been shown to have a beneficial impact on mental health and well-being. Developing and maintaining supportive relationships can help to improve one's general mental health and well-being.

Transcranial magnetic stimulation (TMS) and transcranial direct current stimulation (tDCS) are two brain stimulation techniques being researched as potential ways for improving cognitive function.

To summarize, mind optimization entails a variety of strategies and methods such as mindfulness, meditation, cognitive training, nootropics, sleep, stress management, social support, and brain stimulation. These methods can help to improve overall mental health and well-being by improving cognitive function, reducing stress and anxiety, and improving overall mental health and well-being. As with body optimization, it is critical to use these methods with caution and under the supervision of a healthcare provider.

Tension control

Stress is a natural component of living, but chronic stress can harm both physical and mental health. Stress management is an important aspect of biohacking because it includes the use of strategies and techniques to help manage and reduce stress levels.

Here are some stress-reduction methods that work:

Mindfulness is the practice of paying nonjudgmental attention to the current moment. Individuals who practice mindfulness can become more aware of their thoughts and emotions, as well as learn to react to stressors more productively. Mindfulness has been shown in studies to reduce stress and enhance overall well-being.

Meditation entails focusing one's attention on a specific object, such as the breath, a mantra, or a visualization. Meditation has been shown to reduce stress, anxiety, and depression, as well as enhance overall mental health.

Social support has been shown to have a beneficial impact on mental health and well-being. Building and keeping supportive relationships can aid in stress reduction and overall well-being.

Relaxation methods, such as deep breathing, progressive muscle relaxation, and guided imagery, can aid in stress reduction and relaxation. These techniques are particularly beneficial in times of high stress.

Poor time management can add to high-stress levels. Individuals can reduce stress and feel more in charge of their lives by prioritizing tasks and setting realistic goals.

In conclusion, stress management is an essential aspect of biohacking that entails employing strategies and techniques to manage and reduce stress levels. Mindfulness, meditation, exercise, sleep, social support, relaxation techniques, and time management are all effective stress management tactics. Individuals can improve their overall well-being and ability to manage stress by incorporating these techniques into their everyday routines.

Mindfulness and meditation

Dan Harris, an ABC News journalist and news anchor, has a real-life tale that exemplifies the benefits of meditation and mindfulness. Harris struggled with anxiety and depression in his early work and turned to drugs to deal with them. However, after having a panic attack on live television in 2004, he sought out more healthy coping strategies, such as meditation.

Harris was initially skeptical of meditation, dismissing it as a "weird, hippy-dippy phenomenon." However, he quickly discovered that regular meditation practice helped him manage his anxiety and improve his overall well-being. Harris went on to publish "10% Happier," a book that details his journey to meditation and mindfulness and how it has helped him become more resilient and productive.

Through his experience with meditation and mindfulness, Harris learned several valuable lessons. First, he learned that it is possible to alter your thought patterns and become more conscious of your mental state.

He discovered that by practicing mindfulness, he was better able to manage his stress levels and capture negative thoughts and emotions before they spiraled out of control. Second, Harris discovered that meditation is a long-term practice that requires devotion and commitment. He discovered that the benefits of meditation were not instantaneous, but accumulated over time as he practiced and refined his technique.

Finally, Harris discovered that meditation and awareness are not "one-size-fits-all" practices. He discovered that various techniques and approaches worked for different people, and it was critical to figure out what worked best for him. Overall, Harris' tale demonstrates the effectiveness of meditation and mindfulness in improving mental health and well-being. It is possible to become more resilient, handle stress, and improve your overall quality of life by committing to regular practice and discovering what works best for you.

Andy Puddicombe, the co-founder of the meditation app Headspace, has another real-life tale that demonstrates the benefits of meditation and mindfulness. As a young adult,

Puddicombe battled with anxiety and depression and turned to meditation to help him manage his mental health. Puddicombe traveled and studied meditation in various nations, including India and Nepal, for several years.
He ultimately became a fully ordained Tibetan Buddhist monk and returned to the United Kingdom to share his meditation knowledge and experience with others.

In 2010, Puddicombe co-founded Headspace intending to make meditation more accessible to a broader audience. Headspace now has over 60 million users globally and provides guided meditation sessions on a variety of subjects such as stress management, sleep, and productivity. Puddicombe has acquired several valuable lessons from his meditation and mindfulness practice.

For starters, he has discovered that mindfulness is not about attempting to attain a specific state of mind, but rather about embracing the present moment as it is. He thinks that acceptance can help reduce stress and anxiety while also improving overall well-being.

Second, Puddicombe has discovered that meditation is more than just sitting in silence and can take many shapes. He encourages people to discover the best meditation practice for them, whether it's mindfulness, visualization, or movement-based meditation.

Finally, Puddicombe considers meditation to be a talent that can be honed over time. He advises people to approach meditation with openness and curiosity and to be patient with themselves as they learn and develop.

Brain improvement

Any technique or practice that seeks to improve cognitive function, such as memory, attention, creativity, and problem-solving, is referred to as cognitive enhancement. While some cognitive enhancement techniques are natural and safe, others require the use of drugs or other substances that may have risks and side effects.

Some of the most common cognitive enhancement techniques are:

Brain training exercises are designed to improve cognitive function by engaging and stimulating specific brain areas. Puzzles, games, and memory training exercises are some examples.

Supplements for nutrition this are supplements, such as omega-3 fatty acids, B vitamins, and ginkgo biloba, have been shown in some studies to enhance cognitive function and brain health.

Nootropic drugs are medications that are specially intended to improve cognitive function. Caffeine, Provigil, and racetams are a few examples. These drugs, however, have potential side effects and should only be used under the supervision of a healthcare expert.

Lifestyle changes: Diet, exercise, and sleep are all factors that can affect cognitive function. Making good changes in these areas can aid in the improvement of cognitive function over time.

Mindfulness and meditation have been shown to improve cognitive function by lowering stress and anxiety, increasing attention and focus, and general well-being.

While cognitive enhancement has the potential to benefit individuals seeking to improve their cognitive function, these methods should be approached with caution. Some techniques, such as nootropic drugs, may pose risks and have side effects.

Before attempting any new technique of cognitive enhancement, it is critical to consult with a healthcare professional. Furthermore, it is critical to emphasize natural and safe methods over potentially risky methods such as drug use, such as brain training exercises, nutritional supplements, and lifestyle changes.

There has been a surge in interest in cognitive enhancement in recent years, especially in the setting of work and academic performance. Many individuals want to improve their cognitive function to increase productivity, creativity, and overall success. However, it is essential to approach cognitive enhancement with skepticism and knowledge.

While some cognitive enhancement techniques are natural and safe, others require the use of drugs or other substances that may have risks and side effects. Caffeine, for example, is a popular and reasonably safe stimulant that can improve cognitive function; however, other nootropic drugs can cause nausea, insomnia, and addiction.

Furthermore, some cognitive enhancement techniques may be ineffective or have limited benefits. Some brain training exercises, for example, may not have long-term effects on a cognitive function beyond the specific activity being trained. As a result, it is critical to approach cognitive enhancement from a holistic standpoint, taking into account a variety of variables that can impact cognitive function, such as diet, exercise, sleep, stress management, and mindfulness.

Adopting healthy lifestyle habits and participating in enjoyable and challenging cognitive stimulation activities can have significant long-term benefits for cognitive function.

Finally, the ethical implications of cognitive enhancement must be considered, especially in the context of social and economic inequality. If cognitive enhancement becomes widespread and only available to those who can afford it, it may exacerbate societal inequalities.

As a result, it is critical to approach cognitive enhancement with an understanding of the potential consequences as well as a commitment to ethical and equitable practices.
Recent research has also highlighted the potential benefits of cognitive enhancement for people suffering from cognitive impairments or neurodegenerative diseases like Alzheimer's.

Certain cognitive training programs, for example, have been shown in some studies to improve cognitive function in older adults and people with mild cognitive impairment. Furthermore, cognitive enhancement techniques such as mindfulness meditation are effective in alleviating symptoms of anxiety, depression, and other mental health conditions. Mindfulness practices entail paying attention to the present moment with openness and non-judgment, and they can aid in the development of emotional resilience and stress management skills.

Overall, cognitive enhancement is a complex and rapidly evolving field with the potential to provide significant benefits to people looking to improve their cognitive function. However, it is important to approach cognitive enhancement with a critical and informed perspective and to prioritize natural and safe methods over potentially risky or ineffective ones. Individuals can improve their cognitive function and general well-being by adopting healthy lifestyle habits, participating in cognitive stimulation activities, and practicing mindfulness.

Nootropics

Nootropics also referred to as "smart drugs," are substances that are said to improve cognitive function, specifically memory, creativity, and motivation. Nootropics are natural or synthetic substances that include herbs, vitamins, minerals, and pharmaceutical drugs.

Certain nootropics have been shown to improve cognitive function. Caffeine, for example, is a common and relatively safe stimulant that can improve alertness and concentration. Furthermore, natural supplements like ginkgo biloba and omega-3 fatty acids have been shown to have potential cognitive benefits.

However, many synthetic nootropics have not been thoroughly researched and may pose risks and side effects. Prescription drugs such as Adderall and Ritalin, for example, have become increasingly popular among students and professionals for cognitive enhancement, but these drugs can have serious side effects such as addiction, anxiety, and insomnia.

Furthermore, the long-term impacts of many nootropics are unknown, and some substances may harm cognitive performance or overall health over time.

As a result, it is critical to proceed with caution when considering nootropics and to emphasize natural and safe methods of cognitive enhancement. Additionally, before using any nootropic supplements or prescription drugs for cognitive enhancement, it is critical to confer with a healthcare expert.

Despite the potential benefits of some nootropics, it is important to remember that cognitive enhancement is a complex and multifaceted process that cannot be achieved solely through supplementation or drug use.

Other factors such as diet, exercise, sleep, stress management, and social support also play important roles in cognitive function and overall well-being.

Moreover, the use of nootropics should not be seen as a substitute for healthy lifestyle habits. While nootropics may offer temporary cognitive benefits, sustainable and long-term cognitive enhancement requires a holistic approach that includes healthy habits and practices.

In addition, the use of nootropics should always be approached with caution, as many substances may have potential risks and side effects. Some synthetic nootropics, for example, have been linked to increased risk of cardiovascular disease, liver damage, and other health problems.

Therefore, it is important to thoroughly research any nootropic supplements or drugs before use and to consult with a healthcare professional to ensure that they are safe and appropriate for individual needs and health conditions.

Overall, while nootropics may offer some potential cognitive benefits, it is important to approach them with caution and to prioritize natural and safe methods of cognitive enhancement. By adopting healthy lifestyle habits and engaging in cognitive stimulation activities, people can enhance their cognitive function and general well-being sustainably and safely.

Chapter four

Tools and Methods for Biohacking

Biohacking is a diverse and quickly changing field that provides individuals seeking to optimize their physical and mental health with a wide range of tools and techniques. The following are some of the most popular and successful biohacking tools and techniques:

Wearable technology: Devices like fitness trackers, smart watches, and heart rate monitors can provide useful data about physical activity, sleep habits, and general health. Individuals can use wearable technology to track their progress, establish goals, and make informed decisions about their lifestyle habits.

Nutrigenomics: This is the study of how food and nutrients combine with genes and affect health. Nutrigenomics testing can assist people in identifying genetic factors that may influence their nutrient needs and making appropriate dietary changes.

Light therapy affects circadian rhythms, which govern sleep patterns and general health.

The use of light-emitting devices such as light boxes, lamps, and glasses to regulate circadian rhythms and enhance sleep quality is known as light therapy.

Cold therapy has been shown to have a variety of health advantages, including reduced inflammation, improved immune function, and improved mental clarity. Techniques such as ice baths, cryotherapy, and cold showers can be used to accomplish cold therapy.

Mindfulness and meditation are practices that involve focusing the mind on the current instant and have been shown to reduce stress, improve mood, and improve cognitive function. To incorporate mindfulness and meditation into daily living, techniques such as breathing exercises, guided meditations, and mindfulness-based stress reduction can be used.

Physical activity regularly can enhance physical health, mental health, and cognitive performance. Biohacking can be accomplished through a variety of exercise methods, including high-intensity interval training, weightlifting, and yoga.

Breathing exercises can help to relieve stress, enhance mental clarity, and encourage relaxation. To improve breathing patterns and boost oxygenation in the body, techniques such as the Wim Hof method, Box breathing, and Pranayama can be used.

Supplements, such as vitamins, minerals, and herbal remedies, can help to enhance physical and mental wellness. However, it is critical to proceed with caution and to consult with a healthcare expert before beginning any new supplement.

Biofeedback is the use of technology to track physiological reactions such as heart rate, blood pressure, and brain waves. Biofeedback can help people become more conscious of their bodies reactions to stress and learn techniques to control these reactions.

Time-restricted eating entails restricting food intake to a specific time window each day, usually 8-12 hours. It has been demonstrated that time-restricted feeding improves metabolic health, reduces inflammation, and improves sleep quality.

Sauna therapy has been linked to a variety of health benefits, including better cardiovascular health, increased immune function, and decreased inflammation. Sauna treatment can be accomplished using either traditional saunas or infrared saunas.

Grounding entails connecting with the earth's inherent electrical charge either by walking barefoot on grass or sand or by using grounding mats or sheets. Grounding has been linked to lower inflammation, better sleep quality, and lower tension.

Journaling: Keeping a journal of one's thoughts, emotions, and experiences can help to reduce stress, increase self-awareness, and improve mental clarity. Journaling can help you reflect on your biohacking practices and track your progress toward your objectives.

Social connection: Participating in social events and developing meaningful relationships can benefit one's mental health and overall well-being. Social support can help to alleviate stress, improve self-esteem, and encourage positive behavior.

Tracking gadgets and wearables

Wearables and tracking gadgets are becoming more popular as biohacking tools. These devices are intended to monitor and track various aspects of health and fitness, providing people with insights into their habits and allowing them to make positive changes.

Fitness trackers, smart watches, heart rate monitors, and sleep tracks are examples of wearables and tracking devices. These devices can track metrics like steps taken, heart rate, sleep quality, and calories expended. Some devices also include sophisticated functions like GPS tracking, blood oxygen monitoring, and stress monitoring. Wearables and tracking devices can collect data that can be used to find areas for improvement in health and fitness, establish goals, and track progress toward these goals. A fitness tracker, for example, may disclose that a person is not reaching their daily step goal, prompting them to increase their physical activity.

Wearables and tracking devices can also be used to improve workouts by giving information such as heart rate, calories expended, and other metrics. Individuals can use this knowledge to fine-tune their workouts for maximum efficiency and effectiveness. Wearables and tracking devices can be used to measure and improve mental health in addition to physical health. A stress tracker, for example, could provide data on a person's stress levels throughout the day, encouraging them to practice stress-reduction methods such as mindfulness or breathing exercises.

Wearables and tracking devices, however, should be used in conjunction with other biohacking techniques such as exercise, nutrition, and mindfulness. Using technology exclusively to enhance health and fitness can result in a narrow focus on metrics rather than overall health and well-being. Prioritizing natural and safe biohacking practices is also essential, as is consulting with a healthcare professional before using any new device or technology.

Biofeedback

Biofeedback is a technique used to enhance physical and mental health by training a person to control involuntary bodily functions. Biofeedback is a technique that includes using sensors to monitor the body's physiological responses to stress and then providing feedback to the person in the form of visual or auditory signals.

This feedback teaches the person how to regulate physiological reactions to stressors such as heart rate, breathing rate, and muscle tension.

Biofeedback methods come in a variety of forms, including:

Electromyography (EMG): EMG is a technique that detects muscle tension and can be used to teach people how to relax their muscles.

Electroencephalography (EEG): EEG is a technique that measures brain waves and can be used to teach people how to regulate their brain activity and improve their mental health.

Galvanic skin response (GSR): GSR monitors the electrical conductance of the skin and can be used to teach people how to manage their stress.

Heart rate variability (HRV): HRV measures the difference in time between heartbeats and can be used to teach people how to regulate their heart rate and reduce stress.

Biofeedback is frequently used to address a wide range of conditions, such as chronic pain, anxiety, and high blood pressure. It can also be used to boost athletic performance and reduce stress in high-pressure circumstances such as public speaking or stage performance.

One of the benefits of biofeedback is that it can be combined with other techniques like mindfulness, meditation, and relaxation exercises to increase their efficacy.

Biofeedback is a non-invasive technique that people of all ages can use to improve their physical and mental well-being.

Biofeedback is successful in a variety of settings, including:

1. Chronic pain management: Biofeedback can teach people how to regulate their pain by reducing muscle tension and increasing relaxation.

2. Anxiety and stress management: By reducing muscle tension and improving relaxation, biofeedback can assist people in learning how to regulate their stress levels.

3. Hypertension: Biofeedback can teach people how to regulate their blood pressure by reducing stress and increasing relaxation.

4. Insomnia: By reducing muscle tension and improving relaxation, biofeedback can assist people in learning how to regulate their sleep patterns.

Attention deficit hyperactivity disorder (ADHD): By showing people how to control their brain waves, biofeedback can help them improve their focus and attention.

Biofeedback can be performed in a clinical environment by a trained healthcare professional or at home using a biofeedback device. Biofeedback devices can be bought online or in specialty stores for a few hundred to several thousand dollars.

While biofeedback is generally thought to be safe, it is critical to use it under the supervision of a trained healthcare expert. Furthermore, it may not be appropriate for everyone, such as those with certain medical problems or pregnant women. Before starting treatment, as with any medical treatment, it is critical to discuss the potential benefits and risks of biofeedback with a healthcare expert.

Cryotherapy

Cryotherapy is a technique in which the body is exposed to extremely cold temperatures for a short amount of time, usually 2 to 4 minutes. The therapy is designed to encourage healing, reduce inflammation, and offer a variety of other health benefits.

Whole-body cryotherapy is the most prevalent type of cryotherapy, in which the individual is exposed to temperatures as low as -140°C (-220°F) in a specially designed cryo-chamber. Endorphins and other hormones are released by the body during therapy, which can boost mood and reduce pain.

There is some proof that cryotherapy has several advantages, including:

- Cryotherapy can decrease inflammation and swelling, which can help with pain relief.
- Cryotherapy has been shown to enhance athletic performance by increasing circulation, which can help with endurance, strength, and recovery.
- Cryotherapy can enhance the appearance of your face by reducing the appearance of wrinkles and blemishes.

- Reduced stress and anxiety: Cryotherapy can help to reduce stress and anxiety levels, which can enhance overall mood and well-being.

While cryotherapy is generally regarded as safe, it is critical to use it under the supervision of a trained healthcare expert. Furthermore, it may not be appropriate for everyone, such as those with certain medical problems or pregnant women. Before starting cryotherapy treatment, as with any medical treatment, it is critical to discuss the potential benefits and risks with a healthcare expert.

Cryotherapy is successful in reducing inflammation in the body, in addition to the benefits mentioned above. Chronic inflammation has been related to a variety of health issues such as heart disease, cancer, and autoimmune disorders. Cryotherapy has also been shown to enhance blood circulation and flow in the body.

This can help to lower the chance of cardiovascular disease, stroke, and other problems. Improved circulation can also aid in the healing and recovery process after an accident.

Weight loss is another possible advantage of cryotherapy. While the evidence is limited, some studies indicate that cryotherapy can help to increase metabolism and burn calories.

When performed by a trained healthcare professional, cryotherapy is usually regarded as safe. However, there are some risks to the treatment, such as frostbite, skin irritation, and other side effects. Before beginning treatment, it is critical to observe the instructions of the healthcare professional performing the therapy and to notify them of any medical conditions or concerns.

Overall, while cryotherapy has potential benefits, more study is required to fully understand its effects on the body and determine its safety and efficacy in treating various health conditions. Before beginning any new treatment, it is critical to speak with a healthcare professional.

Cryotherapy is classified into two types: whole-body cryotherapy and targeted cryotherapy. Whole-body cryotherapy includes brief exposure to cold temperatures in a cryo-chamber, typically for 2 to 4 minutes. Localized cryotherapy entails using a handheld device to apply cold temperatures to a particular area of the body.

Other types of cold therapy, in addition to cryotherapy, can be used to encourage healing and reduce inflammation in the body. Ice packs, icy water immersion, and cold showers are examples of these.

Athletes and fitness enthusiasts frequently use cryotherapy to promote recovery and reduce muscle soreness after strenuous workouts.

People with chronic pain, arthritis, and other inflammatory diseases also use it. While cryotherapy has possible benefits, it should be noted that it is not a replacement for medical treatment. It should be used as an adjunct therapy under the supervision of a healthcare expert. Furthermore, cryotherapy may not be appropriate for everyone, such as those with certain medical problems or pregnant women.

Overall, cryotherapy is a promising therapy with the potential to benefit a wide variety of medical conditions. More research, however, is required to completely comprehend its effects on the body and determine its long-term safety and effectiveness. Before beginning any new treatment or therapy, it is critical to confer with a healthcare professional.

Photobiomodulation

Photobiomodulation (PBM) is a therapeutic method that uses low-level light to stimulate cellular function and promote healing in the body. PBM usually employs light in the red to near-infrared spectrum, with wavelengths ranging from 600 to 1000 nanometers.

PBM functions by penetrating the skin and being absorbed by mitochondria, our cells' energy-producing powerhouses.

When the mitochondria absorb light, it increases the production of ATP (adenosine triphosphate), which is our cells' main energy source. This increased energy generation can aid in the promotion of healing and the reduction of inflammation in the body.

PBM is successful in the treatment of a variety of medical conditions, including chronic pain, sports injuries, and skin disorders. It is also being researched for its possible use in the treatment of neurological diseases such as Alzheimer's and Parkinson's. PBM can be delivered via several devices, such as handheld devices, helmets, and full-body panels. The procedure is usually painless and non-invasive, and there are no known severe side effects.

One of the benefits of PBM is that it can be combined with other therapies, such as physical therapy, to improve their efficacy. PBM has been shown to increase muscle recovery and pain after exercise, which can help athletes perform better. Overall, PBM is a promising therapy that can benefit a variety of health conditions.

More research, however, is required to completely comprehend its effects on the body and determine its long-term safety and effectiveness. Before beginning any new treatment or therapy, it is critical to confer with a healthcare professional.

In addition to its therapeutic applications, PBM has also been researched for its possible benefits in improving cognitive function and reducing the chance of neurodegenerative diseases. Studies have shown that PBM can increase cerebral blood flow and oxygenation, which can improve cognitive function and lower the chance of dementia.

PBM has also been shown to have anti-inflammatory properties, which may aid in the prevention of chronic illnesses such as heart disease and cancer. PBM was found to reduce inflammation and improve insulin sensitivity in people with type 2 diabetes in one trial. PBM has another potential application in the area of aesthetics. PBM has been shown to increase collagen production, which can help improve skin texture and minimize wrinkle appearance. It's also used to address acne and other skin problems.

While PBM is usually considered safe and well-tolerated, using PBM devices requires caution. PBM overuse or abuse can result in side effects such as skin irritation or burns. Before using PBM devices, it is critical to observe the manufacturer's instructions and consult with a healthcare professional. PBM is a promising therapy with numerous uses. PBM has shown promise in improving cognitive function, reducing inflammation, and promoting healing in the body, but more research is required to completely understand its effects on the body. Before starting PBM treatment, as with any therapy or treatment, it is critical to consult with a healthcare professional.

Another possible application for PBM is in sports efficiency. PBM has been shown to improve muscle recovery and decrease muscle fatigue after exercise. Athletes who got PBM treatment had less muscle soreness and recovered faster than those who did not receive PBM treatment, according to one research.

PBM has also been investigated for its use in the treatment of depression and other mental health problems. PBM has been shown in studies to increase the production of neurotransmitters such as serotonin and dopamine, which can improve mood and decrease depression symptoms.

PBM is being researched for its potential to improve athletic performance and cognitive function in healthy people, in addition to its therapeutic uses. Some athletes and biohackers have begun to use PBM devices to improve their physical and mental efficiency.

While the potential benefits of PBM are intriguing, it is important to note that research in this field is still in its early stages. More research is required to fully comprehend PBM's effects on the body and mind.

It's also worth noting that PBM isn't a replacement for traditional medical therapies. Before using PBM devices, consult with a healthcare professional if you have a medical condition or are having symptoms. Overall, PBM is a promising therapy with a wide variety of possible applications in health, fitness, and wellness.

As research in this field advances, we can expect to learn more about the potential benefits of PBM and its role in optimizing the body and mind.

Reduction of EMF radiation

Our exposure to electromagnetic fields increases as technology becomes more integrated into our everyday lives (EMFs). EMFs are emitted by electronic devices such as mobile phones, laptop computers, and Wi-Fi routers, and a study suggests that prolonged exposure to high levels of EMFs may be harmful to one's health. While it is not possible to fully avoid EMF exposure, steps can be taken to minimize exposure and mitigate potential health risks.

Here are some suggestions for lowering EMF exposure:

- Limit the amount of time you spend on your mobile phone each day, and make calls using a headset or speakerphone.

- When you're not actively using your phone, put it in airplane mode to minimize EMF emissions.

- Sleeping with electronic gadgets is not recommended: Keep electronic devices, particularly those that emit high levels of EMFs, such as laptops and mobile phones, out of the bedroom.

- When using electrical devices, keep them as far away from your body as possible. Use a laptop stand, for example, or put your phone in a bag or purse rather than your pocket.

- Make use of physical connections: When feasible, connect to the internet via wired connections rather than Wi-Fi. This can help to minimize your Wi-Fi radiation exposure.

- There are products on the market that promise to reduce EMF exposure, such as EMF-blocking phone cases or home shielding materials. However, the efficacy of these items is not always obvious.

- Educate yourself and your family about EMFs and how to minimize your exposure to them. Keep up with the newest research and developments in this field.

While reducing EMF exposure may have potential health benefits, more research is required to completely understand the long-term effects of EMF exposure on human health. As a result, if you are concerned about EMF exposure and its potential impact on your health, it is always a good idea to confer with a healthcare expert.

Thermogenesis in the cold

Cold thermogenesis is a biohacking method in which the body is exposed to cold temperatures to elicit a variety of physiological responses. This can be accomplished through activities such as taking cold showers, taking ice baths, or even being exposed to cold conditions. Cold thermogenesis works by triggering the body's natural reaction to cold, which includes thermogenesis. This is the production of heat within the body, which can stimulate the immune system, raise metabolic rate, and improve circulation. Cold exposure has also been shown to boost the production of brown adipose tissue, also known as "brown fat," a type of fat that burns calories to produce heat.

Cold thermogenesis may have the following advantages:

- Cold temperatures can boost your metabolic rate, allowing you to burn more calories and lose weight.
- Cold exposure has been shown to reduce inflammation in the body, which has been linked to a variety of health issues such as heart disease, diabetes, and arthritis.
- Cold exposure can activate the immune system, resulting in a stronger and more resilient immune reaction.
- Improved circulation and oxygenation: Cold thermogenesis can improve circulation and oxygenation, resulting in greater energy and mental clarity.

It's important to note that cold thermogenesis can be unpleasant, particularly at first. To prevent injury, it is critical to begin slowly and progressively increase exposure to cold temperatures. It's also critical to consult with a healthcare professional before embarking on any new health regimen, particularly if you have any underlying health issues.

Chapter five

Biohacking for Life

Biohacking for longevity is a branch of science that focuses on using various techniques and practices to increase human lifespan and general health span. While some of these practices are still being studied and developed, several biohacking strategies have been demonstrated to promote longevity and healthy aging.

Caloric restriction is a dietary strategy in which caloric intake is reduced without creating malnutrition. Caloric restriction has been shown in studies to improve lifespan and delay the onset of age-related diseases.

Intermittent fasting is a dietary practice that includes alternate times of eating and fasting. This practice has been shown to enhance metabolic health, reduce inflammation, and increase lifespan.

Exercise has been shown to increase longevity by improving cardiovascular health, reducing inflammation, and raising mitochondrial function.

Studies have shown that sauna therapy improves cardiovascular performance, reduces inflammation, and promotes longevity.

Anti-aging methods

Anti-aging strategies are a collection of practices and routines aimed at slowing or reversing the aging process and promoting healthy aging. Here are some anti-aging techniques that work:

Eating a healthy diet rich in whole foods, fruits and vegetables, lean proteins, and healthy fats can provide the body with important nutrients and antioxidants, slowing the aging process.

Stress Management: Chronic stress can hasten age and raise the chance of age-related diseases. Meditation, yoga, and deep breathing are effective stress management techniques that can help reduce stress and support healthy aging.

Sleep: Getting enough sleep is critical for good aging. The body repairs and regenerates tissues while sleeping, and a lack of sleep has been related to an increased chance of chronic diseases.

Sun protection: Sun exposure can hasten the aging process and increase the chance of skin cancer. Sunscreen, clothing, and averting direct sunlight during peak hours can all help to slow down the aging process.

Toxin Avoidance: Toxins, such as tobacco smoke, air pollution, and chemicals, can hasten to age and increase the chance of chronic diseases. Toxin reduction can help support healthy aging.

Hormone Replacement Therapy: Hormone replacement treatment can help restore hormone levels and alleviate symptoms of menopause and andropause, improving quality of life and promoting healthy aging.

Mental stimulation, such as acquiring a new skill or playing brain games, can improve cognitive function and encourage healthy aging.

Maintaining social ties can help reduce stress and depression and improve overall well-being, promoting healthy aging.

Telomere extension

Telomeres are the protective caps that form at the ends of our chromosomes as we mature. Telomere lengthening is the process of lengthening these protective caps to delay or even reverse the aging process.

Here are some strategies for promoting telomere lengthening:

- Adopting a healthy lifestyle, which includes regular exercise, a nutritious diet, and stress management, can help support telomere lengthening.
- Certain dietary supplements, such as vitamin D, omega-3 fatty acids, and antioxidants, have been shown to support telomere lengthening.
- Telomerase Activators: Telomerase is an enzyme that supports the lengthening of telomeres. Astragalus root and cycloastragenol, for example, have been shown to activate telomerase and encourage telomere lengthening.
- Meditation and mindfulness practice has been shown in studies to support telomere lengthening by reducing stress and improving overall well-being.

- Fasting: It has been shown that intermittent fasting or periodic fasting promotes telomere lengthening by triggering cellular repair mechanisms.

Certain lifestyle modification programs, such as the Telomere Effect program created by Dr. Elizabeth Blackburn and Elissa Epel, encourage healthy lifestyle habits and stress management techniques to promote telomere lengthening.

One study published in the journal Rejuvenation Research in 2016 looked at how a complete lifestyle intervention program affected telomere length in a group of healthy males. A plant-based diet, frequent exercise, stress-reduction techniques, and social support were all part of the program.

After 5 years, males in the intervention group had significantly longer telomeres than men in the control group who did not take part in the lifestyle intervention. Another research published in the journal aging in 2017 looked at how a 3-month lifestyle intervention program affected telomere length in a group of overweight and obese women.

A low-calorie diet, moderate exercise, and stress-reduction techniques were all part of the regimen.

The findings revealed that women in the training group had significantly longer telomeres than those in the control group.

While these findings indicate that lifestyle interventions may promote telomere lengthening, more research is required to fully comprehend the mechanisms and potential benefits of telomere lengthening for healthy aging. It's essential to note that telomere length is only one factor that contributes to aging; there are likely many others.

Other possible telomere lengthening strategies, such as nutrient and hormone supplementation, have been investigated. However, the evidence for these approaches is murky, and more study is required to determine their efficacy. One research, for example, published in the journal PLoS One in 2014, looked at the effects of a nutritional supplement containing a blend of several vitamins, minerals, and antioxidants on telomere length in a group of middle-aged adults.

The findings revealed that there was a significant increase in telomere length after 6 months of supplementation compared to a control group that did not receive the supplement. However, because this was a small study and the supplement used was a proprietary blend, it's difficult to draw solid conclusions about its efficacy. Another approach being investigated is the use of hormones like growth hormone and dehydroepiandrosterone (DHEA) to encourage telomere lengthening. Some studies have found that these hormones may have a positive effect on telomere length, but the evidence is mixed, and more research is required to completely grasp the potential benefits and risks of telomere-lengthening hormone supplementation.

Overall, while telomere lengthening is an interesting potential strategy for promoting healthy aging, it's critical to proceed with caution and confer with a healthcare expert before experimenting with new supplements or hormones. Furthermore, focusing on lifestyle interventions such as a healthy diet, regular exercise, stress reduction, and good sleep hygiene may be a more long-term and evidence-based strategy to support overall health and longevity.

Fasting and calorie limitation

Caloric restriction and fasting are two common biohacking techniques that have been shown to improve longevity and health. Caloric restriction is the practice of lowering calorie intake while keeping adequate nutrition. It has been shown in animal models such as mice and rats to increase lifespan and enhance health. Caloric restriction has been shown in humans to enhance aging biomarkers such as insulin sensitivity, inflammation, and oxidative stress. Long-term caloric restriction, on the other hand, can be difficult to maintain and, if not carefully watched, can lead to malnutrition.

Intermittent fasting (IF) is a type of fasting in which times of fasting are alternated with periods of normal eating. The 16/8 method, in which an individual fast for 16 hours and consumes during an 8-hour window, and the 5:2 method, in which an individual eats normally for 5 days and restricts calories to 500-600 on two non-consecutive days, are two popular IF protocols. In terms of improving biomarkers of aging and lowering the risk of chronic diseases such as diabetes and cardiovascular disease, IF is comparable to caloric restriction.

Extended fasting, in which a person fasts for 24 hours or more, is another type of fasting that has acquired popularity in recent years. Extensive fasting has been shown in animal studies to have powerful effects on health and longevity, including increasing lifespan and lowering the chance of cancer and other chronic diseases. More research is required, however, to completely understand the potential benefits and risks of prolonged fasting in humans. Caloric restriction and fasting, in general, are promising biohacking techniques for promoting longevity and health. However, it is critical to proceed with caution and collaborate with a healthcare professional to ensure adequate nutrition is kept and any possible risks are monitored.

Caloric restriction and fasting are two effective anti-aging techniques. Caloric restriction entails lowering overall calorie intake while keeping sufficient nutrition. Fasting is the practice of limiting or eliminating calorie intake for a set amount of time. Both methods have been shown to increase longevity and overall health. Caloric restriction has been investigated in a variety of animal models and has been shown to prolong life and delay the onset of age-related diseases such as cancer, diabetes, and cardiovascular disease. Caloric restriction has been shown in humans to increase insulin sensitivity, reduce inflammation, and boost cardiovascular health markers.

Fasting has also been shown to have anti-aging benefits. Intermittent fasting has been shown in studies to increase insulin sensitivity, reduce inflammation, and promote autophagy, the body's natural process of cellular cleanup and repair. Fasting has also been shown to boost growth hormone production, which is important for cellular repair and regeneration.

Fasting can be divided into three types: time-restricted feeding, alternate-day fasting, and prolonged fasting. Time-restricted feeding entails restricting food intake to a specific time window each day, usually 8-10 hours. Alternate-day fasting entails alternating between days of regular eating and days of calorie restriction. Prolonged fasting is defined as fasting for 24 hours or more.

While caloric restriction and fasting can have significant health benefits, these strategies should be used with caution and under the supervision of a healthcare expert.

Calorie restriction or fasting can be difficult and may not be suitable for everyone. It is also critical to ensure that nutrient requirements are fulfilled, as well as that any medications or medical conditions are taken into account.

Overall, caloric restriction and fasting are effective ways to promote health and life. Individuals may be able to improve insulin sensitivity, reduce inflammation, and promote cellular repair and regeneration by decreasing overall calorie consumption or fasting for specific periods.

Hormone balancing

Hormone optimization is an important aspect of biohacking that entails detecting hormonal imbalances and applying lifestyle changes, supplements, or medications to restore hormonal balance. Hormones are chemical messengers that control a variety of bodily processes such as metabolism, growth, mood, sexual function, and stress reaction. Hormonal imbalances can cause a variety of health problems, including weight increase, fatigue, mood swings, sleep disruptions, and a loss of libido. Biohackers frequently use hormone optimization to improve their general health and well-being.

Testosterone, which promotes muscle growth, bone density, and sex drive in men, is one of the most commonly optimized hormones. Although testosterone levels naturally decline as men age, lifestyle factors such as diet and exercise can also influence testosterone production. To boost testosterone levels and enhance physical performance, biohackers may use supplements or medications.

Another hormone that can be improved through biohacking is estrogen. Estrogen is essential for women's menstrual period regulation and bone health. Excess estrogen, on the other hand, can raise the risk of breast cancer and other health problems. To optimize estrogen levels and maintain hormonal balance, biohackers may use supplements or make lifestyle adjustments. Growth hormone, thyroid hormone, and cortisol are other hormones that can be improved through biohacking. The thyroid hormone regulates metabolism and energy levels, whereas the growth hormone is required for muscle development and repair.

Cortisol, also known as the "stress hormone," can be elevated in reaction to chronic stress. Biohackers may use supplements or make changes to their lifestyle to regulate cortisol levels and minimize the negative impacts of stress on their health.

Hormone optimization is an important part of biohacking because it can help people improve their general health and well-being. Biohackers can improve their physical and mental performance, lower their risk of chronic disease, and possibly even extend their lifespan by identifying and correcting hormonal imbalances.

However, when implementing any hormonal optimization strategies, it is critical to work with a qualified healthcare professional, as hormonal imbalances can have severe health consequences if not addressed correctly.

Hormone optimization is an essential aspect of longevity biohacking. Our bodies natural hormone production declines as we age, resulting in a decline in physical and cognitive function.

Hormones regulate numerous bodily processes, including metabolism, energy generation, mood, and immune function. We can slow the aging process and enhance overall health and longevity by optimizing hormone levels through biohacking.

One common hormone optimization approach is to supplement with bio identical hormones, which are structurally identical to the hormones produced naturally by the body. BHRT is commonly used to treat menopausal symptoms in women, but it can also be used to optimize hormone levels in both males and women.

Diet and lifestyle adjustments are another way to optimize hormones. Certain foods, such as cruciferous vegetables and flaxseeds, contain hormone-balancing compounds. Regular exercise, stress management techniques and adequate sleep can all aid in hormone regulation.

Testosterone optimization is a common focus for male hormone optimization. Testosterone is essential for muscle mass, bone density, and overall vitality. However, testosterone levels naturally decline as people get older. Strength training, intermittent fasting, and supplementation with certain vitamins and minerals are all biohacking techniques that can help increase testosterone levels naturally. Similarly, estrogen optimization is a critical factor for women. Estrogen is involved in the regulation of bone density, cognitive performance, and cardiovascular health. Strength training and incorporating phytoestrogen-rich foods into the diet are two biohacking methods that can help women optimize their estrogen levels.

Thyroid function optimization is also important for total hormone optimization. Hormones produced by the thyroid gland control metabolism, energy production, and body temperature. Biohacking methods such as iodine and selenium supplementation, adequate sleep, and stress management can all help optimize thyroid function.

To summarize, hormone optimization is a critical component of biohacking for life. We can improve general health and extend our lifespan by taking bio identical hormones, making dietary and lifestyle changes, and incorporating biohacking methods to optimize specific hormones. When employing hormone optimization strategies, it is critical to collaborate with a qualified healthcare practitioner because improper hormone levels can have negative health consequences.

Chapter six

Biohacking for Disease Prevention and Therapy

Biohacking is a broad term that refers to a variety of techniques and behaviors used to improve human health and performance. Disease prevention and treatment is an important aspects of biohacking, and many biohackers use various tools and methods to reduce their risk of getting common chronic illnesses such as cancer, heart disease, and diabetes.

A healthy diet is essential for avoiding chronic illness. Biohackers may use tools such as food monitoring apps to ensure they get enough nutrients while avoiding unhealthy foods.

They may also try various diets, such as low-carb or ketogenic diets, to see what works best for their systems.

Regular exercise is also beneficial for illness prevention. Biohackers may use tools such as fitness trackers to measure their activity levels and optimize their workouts.

Sleep is critical for overall health, and biohackers may use tools such as sleep trackers to ensure they are receiving enough rest.

They may also try various sleep aids and methods to improve the quality of their sleep, such as meditation or light therapy.

Optimizing gut health and microbiota

The gut microbiome is a community of microorganisms found in the human digestive system that plays an important role in general health and well-being. In recent years, the study has shown that a healthy microbiome can help prevent and even treat a variety of diseases.

Biohacking techniques can be used to enhance gut health and microbiome.

Dietary changes, supplementation, and lifestyle changes are examples of these methods.

Dietary changes are one of the most effective methods to improve gut health. A diet high in whole, unprocessed foods and low in sugar and refined carbohydrates has been shown in studies to promote gut health. This is because these foods provide the nutrients that the gut microbiome requires to flourish. The use of probiotics and prebiotics is another essential factor in gut health.

Probiotics are live bacteria that help populate the stomach with beneficial microorganisms, whereas prebiotics is the fiber that feeds these bacteria. Including fermented vegetables, kefir, and yogurt in your diet can provide a natural supply of probiotics. Foods containing prebiotics include scallions, garlic, bananas, and oats.

Aside from dietary adjustments, lifestyle changes such as stress management and regular exercise can also help to improve gut health. Regular exercise has been shown to enhance gut diversity and function while stress has been shown to disrupt the gut microbiome. Overall, improving gut health through biohacking techniques has the potential to have a significant effect on overall health and well-being. Simple dietary and lifestyle changes can improve gut diversity and function, resulting in a healthier, happier existence.

The gut microbiome is a microbial community that lives in our digestive system. These microorganisms are important for digestion, immunity, and general health.

A recent study has revealed that the health of our gut microbiome is closely related to a variety of health problems, including obesity, type 2 diabetes, autoimmune disorders, and even mental health.

Biohacking methods for gut health and microbiome optimization include:

Eating a variety of whole foods: Eating a diverse range of whole foods, particularly plant-based foods, can aid in the growth and diversity of beneficial gut bacteria.

Avoiding processed foods and sugary drinks: Processed foods and added sugars can upset the gut bacteria balance, resulting in inflammation and other health issues.

Utilization of probiotics and prebiotics: Probiotics are live bacteria that can help replenish beneficial gut bacteria, whereas prebiotics is fibers that these bacteria can feed on.

Stress management: Because chronic stress can disrupt the balance of gut bacteria, stress reduction techniques like meditation, yoga, and deep breathing can help support gut health.

Regular exercise has been shown to have a positive impact on the gut microbiome, promoting the growth of beneficial bacteria.

Adequate sleep is essential for overall health, including the health of the gut microbiome.

Avoiding unnecessary antibiotics: Because antibiotics can upset the balance of gut bacteria, they should be used only when strictly essential.

Defense system booster

Biohacking can be used to boost the immune system and decrease disease risk. Because the immune system is so important in defending the body against sickness and illness, it must be kept in peak condition. Here are some biohacking methods for improving the immune system:

Nutrition: A well-balanced diet rich in fruits and vegetables, lean protein, and healthy fats can aid to strengthen the immune system. Eating foods rich in vitamins and minerals, such as vitamin C and zinc, can also help. Consuming processed meals, sugar, and unhealthy fats, on the other hand, can impair the immune system.

Exercise: Regular physical exercise can boost the immune system by lowering inflammation and stress. Moderate exercise for 30 minutes a day, five times a week, such as brisk walking or cycling, can boost immune function.

Sleep: Adequate sleep is essential for the immune system to operate properly. Sleep deprivation can weaken the immune system and raise the risk of infection.

Stress management: Because chronic stress can harm the immune system, it is critical to keep stress under control. Meditation, yoga, deep breathing, and other relaxation methods can help you reduce stress and boost your immune system.

Medications, such as probiotics, vitamin D, and omega-3 fatty acids, can help boost the immune system. Probiotics can help promote gut health, which is important for immune function, and vitamin D and omega-3 fatty acids are anti-inflammatory.

Exposure to cold: Cold temperatures, such as having cold showers or immersing in ice baths, can stimulate and improve the immune system's function.

Management of chronic diseases

Biohacking can also be used as an adjunct treatment for chronic illnesses. Chronic diseases, such as diabetes, heart disease, and autoimmune disorders, are conditions that last a long time and usually advance slowly. While conventional medicine focuses on treating the symptoms of chronic diseases, biohacking can aid in the treatment of the underlying causes. Optimizing diet and nutrition is one of the most important methods to manage chronic diseases through biohacking. A diet rich in anti-inflammatory foods, for example, can help manage autoimmune disorders and lower the risk of heart disease. Similarly, a low-carbohydrate diet can aid in the management of diabetes by lowering blood sugar levels.

Exercise and fitness can also help with the management of chronic diseases. Regular exercise, for example, can improve insulin sensitivity in diabetics and lower the risk of heart disease. By increasing bone density, resistance training can aid in the management of osteoporosis. Stress management methods, such as meditation and mindfulness, can also help manage chronic diseases.

Chronic stress has been linked to a broad variety of health problems, including heart disease, diabetes, and depression. Individuals can reduce their risk of developing chronic diseases and improve their overall health by managing their stress levels.

Furthermore, by optimizing sleep and rest, biohacking can aid in the management of chronic diseases. Chronic diseases frequently disrupt sleep habits and cause fatigue, making management challenging. Individuals can reduce their chance of acquiring chronic diseases and manage the symptoms of existing conditions by improving their sleep quality and duration.

Supplementation can also help with the management of chronic illnesses. Omega-3 fatty acid supplements, for example, can help reduce inflammation and control the symptoms of autoimmune disorders. Vitamin D supplements can help individuals with osteoporosis improve their bone health.

Finally, by optimizing the microbiome and immune system, biohacking can be used to control chronic diseases.

Prebiotics and probiotics, for example, can help enhance gut health and reduce inflammation, which can aid in the management of autoimmune disorders. Immune-boosting supplements like elderberry and Echinacea can help decrease the severity and frequency of colds and flu.

In conclusion, biohacking can be used as a complementary strategy to chronic disease management. Individuals can improve their general health and manage the symptoms of chronic diseases by optimizing food and nutrition, exercise and fitness, stress management, sleep and rest, supplementation, and the microbiome and immune system.

Management of chronic diseases

Chronic disease control is an important component of biohacking. Chronic diseases are long-term conditions that can significantly reduce a person's quality of life. Heart disease, diabetes, cancer, and autoimmune disorders are examples of chronic diseases.

Biohacking can be used to treat chronic diseases in a variety of ways. One approach is to use lifestyle changes to reduce the risk of chronic disease development in the first place. This can include improving diet and exercise, reducing stress, and avoiding environmental toxins. Biohacking can be used to manage symptoms and enhance overall health in people who have already been diagnosed with a chronic disease. This can include taking specific supplements, making dietary changes, and using advanced testing to track progress and modify treatment plans as needed.

Using a continuous glucose monitoring (CGM) system to control diabetes is one example of biohacking for chronic disease management. CGM systems use a small sensor placed beneath the skin to constantly measure glucose levels.

This enables diabetics to monitor their glucose levels in real-time and adjust their diet and medication to maintain their levels within a healthy range.

Another case in point is the use of biofeedback techniques to control chronic pain. Monitoring bodily functions such as heart rate and muscle tension and using feedback to learn how to regulate those functions is what biofeedback is all about. Individuals with chronic pain conditions can use this to reduce pain and enhance their overall quality of life.

In conclusion, chronic disease management is an important element of biohacking. Biohacking can be used to prevent chronic diseases, manage symptoms, and improve general health in people who have already been diagnosed. Individuals can take charge of their health and enhance their quality of life by implementing targeted lifestyle changes, supplements, and advanced testing.

Medicine that regenerates itself

Regenerative medicine is a branch of medicine that uses various methods to restore the function and structure of damaged or diseased tissues and organs. To encourage tissue regeneration and repair, stem cells, growth factors, and other biomolecules may be used.

One of the primary objectives of regenerative medicine is to reduce the need for organ transplantation by developing novel therapies that can aid in the healing and regeneration of damaged tissues and organs. One of the most promising approaches to achieving this objective is stem cell therapy. Stem cells are special cells in the body that can differentiate into different kinds of cells and can be used to replace or repair damaged tissues.

The development of tissue engineering techniques is another significant area of regenerative medicine. This entails creating artificial tissues and organs that can be implanted into the body using specialty biomaterials and 3D printing technologies. This method has great potential for treating a wide range of diseases and injuries, including heart disease, diabetes, and spinal cord injuries.

There are also several other approaches to regenerative medicine, including gene therapy and the use of growth factors and other molecules to stimulate tissue regeneration. While the field is still relatively new, there is growing interest in regenerative medicine among researchers and healthcare professionals, and there is hope that these approaches will lead to new treatments for a wide range of diseases and conditions.

Regenerative medicine is an emerging field of biomedicine that aims to replace, repair, or regenerate damaged or diseased tissues and organs by harnessing the body's natural healing processes.

It marks a paradigm change in healthcare, moving away from treating symptoms and towards restoring function by repairing and replacing damaged cells, tissues, and organs.

The ultimate aim of regenerative medicine is to create treatments that can not only restore lost function, but also prevent or cure chronic diseases such as heart disease, diabetes, and neurodegenerative disorders. This is accomplished through a range of innovative technologies, including stem cells, gene therapy, tissue engineering, and biomaterials.

One of the most promising fields of regenerative medicine is stem cell therapy. Stem cells are unique cells that can differentiate into any type of cell in the body, making them a potent tool for repairing and replacing damaged tissues. Stem cells can be obtained from several sources, including embryonic tissue, adult tissue, and cord blood. Researchers are investigating the use of stem cells to cure a variety of conditions such as heart disease, stroke, diabetes, and spinal cord injuries.

Tissue engineering, which involves growing new tissues or organs in the lab and then transplanting them into the body, is another important field of regenerative medicine.

This approach has the potential to transform the treatment of conditions such as organ failure, where donor organs are in short supply for transplantation. Tissue engineering is the process of combining cells, biomaterials, and growth factors to form a scaffold that can support the growth and development of new tissue.

Gene therapy is another promising method in regenerative medicine, involving the use of DNA to treat or prevent disease. Gene therapy can be used to replace or repair faulty genes, or to introduce new genes that can help to prevent or cure illness. Researchers are presently exploring the use of gene therapy to treat a variety of conditions, including cystic fibrosis, sickle cell disease, and inherited forms of blindness.

Finally, biomaterials are playing an increasingly essential part in regenerative medicine. Biomaterials are synthetic or natural substances that can be used to substitute or heal damaged tissues. They can be used to make scaffolds for tissue engineering, as well as to deliver drugs or growth factors to the body.

Researchers are currently working on a variety of novel biomaterials, such as hydrogels, nanofibers, and 3D-printed structures. While regenerative medicine is still in its infancy, it has the potential to revolutionize how we treat and prevent disease. By harnessing the body's natural healing mechanisms, regenerative medicine offers the promise of not only restoring lost function but also preventing chronic diseases from developing in the first place. As research in this field continues to advance, we can expect to see increasingly sophisticated and effective treatments that offer hope to millions of people around the world.

Biohacking Ethics and Hazards

Regenerative medicine is a branch of medicine that uses various methods to restore the function and structure of damaged or diseased tissues and organs. To encourage tissue regeneration and repair, stem cells, growth factors, and other biomolecules may be used.

One of the primary objectives of regenerative medicine is to reduce the need for organ transplantation by developing novel therapies that can aid in the healing and regeneration of damaged tissues and organs.

One of the most promising approaches to achieving this objective is stem cell therapy. Stem cells are special cells in the body that can differentiate into different kinds of cells and can be used to replace or repair damaged tissues.

The development of tissue engineering techniques is another significant area of regenerative medicine. This entails creating artificial tissues and organs that can be implanted into the body using specialty biomaterials and 3D printing technologies.

This method has great potential for treating a wide variety of diseases and injuries, including heart disease, diabetes, and spinal cord injuries.

Gene therapy and the use of growth factors and other molecules to stimulate tissue regeneration are two other approaches to regenerative medicine. While the field is still in its early stages, there is increasing interest in regenerative medicine among researchers and healthcare professionals, with the hope that these methods will lead to new treatments for a variety of illnesses and conditions.

Regenerative medicine is a new area of biomedicine that uses the body's natural healing processes to replace, repair, or regenerate damaged or diseased tissues and organs. It marks a paradigm change in healthcare, shifting from treating symptoms to restoring function through the repair and replacement of damaged cells, tissues, and organs. The ultimate goal of regenerative medicine is to create treatments that not only restore lost function but also prevent or cure chronic diseases like heart disease, diabetes, and neurodegenerative disorders. This is accomplished through a variety of cutting-edge technologies such as stem cells, gene therapy, tissue engineering, and biomaterials.

Stem cell remedy is one of the most promising areas of regenerative drugs. Stem cells are one-of-a-kind cells that can separate into any type of cell in the body, making them an effective instrument for repairing and replacing damaged apkins. Stem cells can be acquired from several different sources, including embryonic towels, adult towels, and cord blood.

Experimenters are probing the use of stem cells to cure a variety of conditions similar to heart complaints, stroke, diabetes, and spinal cord injuries. Towel engineering, which involves growing new apkins or organs in the lab and also broadcasting them into the body, is another important field of regenerative drugs. This system has the implicit to transfigure the treatment of conditions similar to organ failure, where patron organs are in limited force for transplantation. Towel engineering is the process of combining cells, biomaterials, and growth factors to form an altar that can support the conformation and development of a new towel. Gene remedy, which involves the use of DNA to treat or help complaints, is another promising system in regenerative drugs. Gene remedies can be used to replace or repair defective genes, as well as to introduce new genes that can prop in complaint forestallment or treatment. Gene remedy is presently being delved into for the treatment of a variety of conditions, including cystic fibrosis, sickle cell complaint, and inherited forms of blindness. Eventually, biomaterials are getting more important in regenerative drugs. Biomaterials are substances, either synthetic or natural, that can be used to replace or repair damaged apkins.

They can be used to make pulpits for towel engineering and to deliver medicines or growth factors to the body. Experimenters are presently working on a variety of new biomaterials, similar to hydrogels, nanofibers, and 3D-published structures. While the regenerative drug is still in its immaturity, it has the implicit to revise how we treat and help illness. The regenerative drug holds the pledge of not only restoring lost function but also precluding habitual conditions from developing in the first place by employing the body's natural mending mechanisms. As an exploration in this field advances, we can anticipate seeing more sophisticated and effective treatments that will give a stopgap to millions of people all over the world.

Chapter seven

Biohacking Ethics and Danger

Biohacking is a growing trend in which colorful styles and technologies are used to optimize the body and mind. While there are multitudinous possible advantages to biohacking, there are also ethical and safety enterprises to consider. One of the major ethical enterprises with biohacking is the possibility of inequality.

While numerous biohacking ways and tools are nicely affordable and accessible, some are more precious and exclusive and may be available only to the fat. This could complicate social inequalities by widening the difference between those who have access to these technologies and those who do not. Another ethical issue to consider is the possibility of unintended impacts. While numerous biohacking ways and tools have been completely delved into and are generally regarded as safe, there's still the possibility that they may have negative goods on the body and psyche. Some nootropics, for illustration, have been linked to adverse responses, and there's a threat of dependence or other negative issues associated with their use.

There are safety pitfalls involved with some biohacking ways and tools, in addition to ethical issues. Cryotherapy, for illustration, entails exposing the body to extremely cold temperatures, which can be dangerous if not done rightly. Also, some supplements and nootropics can interact with other specifics, conceivably performing adverse responses. It's essential to note that numerous of the pitfalls associated with biohacking can be reduced by conducting thorough exploration, consulting with healthcare experts, and using biohacking tools and ways responsibly. Still, it's critical to be conscious of the pitfalls and approach biohacking with caution and awareness.

To epitomize, while biohacking has the implicit to give multitudinous advantages for optimizing the body and mind, it's critical to approach it with caution and regard for ethical and safety enterprises. Individualities can safely and responsibly probe the world of biohacking and optimize their health and good by being apprehensive of these pitfalls and taking measures to alleviate them. Pitfalls and prices must be balanced. Biohacking is the practice of experimenting on oneself to ameliorate one's health and effectiveness. While biohacking has multitudinous advantages, it also has pitfalls that must be counted against the possible advantages. Before trying any biohacking system, it's critical to exercise caution and weigh the pitfalls and benefits.

Adverse responses to supplements, adverse responses to nootropics, infection from biohacking procedures, and injury from physical biohacking styles are some of the pitfalls involved with biohacking. There's also the possibility of psychic detriment, similar to an unhealthy obsession with one's health or a negative body image. To reduce the pitfalls of biohacking, it's critical to completely study the ways, gain professional guidance, and precisely cover one's progress.

It's also critical to begin sluggishly and make up the intensity of biohacking styles. The ethical ramifications of biohacking must also be considered when balancing pitfalls and benefits. Biohacking entails experimenting on oneself, and it's debatable whether people have the legal right to do so. There are also enterprises about biohacking's implicit effect on society and the terrain. Supplements and nootropics, for illustration, can give people an illegal advantage over those who don't use them. Likewise, some biohacking styles may have environmental consequences, similar as using too important energy or producing waste.

To address the ethical implications of biohacking, it is necessary to consider the possible societal and environmental consequences. It is also critical to respect people's autonomy and rights while ensuring that they do not harm themselves or others.

To summarize, biohacking has numerous benefits, but it also has risks that must be weighed against the possible benefits. To reduce the risks of biohacking, it is critical to thoroughly study techniques, obtain professional advice, and carefully monitor progress. Furthermore, the ethical implications of biohacking must be considered, and measures must be taken to address any possible negative effects on society and the environment.

In any biohacking practice, balancing risks and advantages is critical. To determine whether a specific intervention or practice is worthwhile, it is critical to weigh the possible risks against the benefits. On the one hand, some biohacks may provide substantial health, performance, and well-being benefits. Certain supplements, for example, omega-3 fatty acids, have been shown to lower the chance of heart disease and stroke.

Similarly, regular exercise can help avoid several chronic diseases, including diabetes and cancer, as well as improve physical and mental health.

Every biohack, however, entails some level of risk. Excessive supplementation, for example, can result in toxicity and other negative side effects. Intense exercise can also cause harm if it is not done properly or if the body is not properly rested and recovered. Furthermore, some biohacking techniques, such as self-experimentation with untested compounds, may pose unknown risks that cannot be fully assessed.

As a result, when contemplating a biohacking practice, it is critical to conduct extensive research and confer with qualified experts to determine the potential risks and benefits. It is also critical to heed your body and keep an eye out for any negative effects. If a hack is causing harm or pain, it should be stopped immediately.

Finally, the key to balancing risks and benefits is to proceed with caution, care, and educated decision-making when it comes to biohacking. Individuals can improve their health and well-being while minimizing possible harm by doing so.

Judicial implications

Biohacking is a new subject, and the legal landscape surrounding it is still developing. As a consequence, determining what is legal and what is not can be difficult. Some biohacking techniques are legal, while others are illegal or unethical.

Biohacking frequently involves the use of substances and technologies that have not been authorized by regulatory bodies such as the FDA. Some people, for example, may use unapproved drugs or supplements to improve their brain function or physical performance. Others may change their genetic makeup using gene-editing technologies such as

CRISPR. While these practices may have some advantages, they may also be hazardous to one's health and well-being.

Biohacking raises concerns about privacy and informed consent, in addition to the risks involved with the use of unapproved substances and technologies. The use of wearable devices to gather personal health data, for example, raises concerns about who has access to that data and how it is used.

Individuals interested in biohacking should be conscious of the legal and ethical implications of their actions. Seeking the advice of a medical professional or a legal expert can assist people in making informed choices about their biohacking practices while reducing the risk of negative consequences. Furthermore, policymakers must consider the implications of biohacking and create regulations that safeguard the public while allowing for innovation and advancement in the field.

Conclusion

Finally, biohacking is a new field that aims to improve human performance and health through the use of various tools, techniques, and lifestyle interventions. Biohackers want to take control of their biology to improve physical and mental health, avoid illness, and live longer. They employ a variety of methods, including food and nutrition, exercise and fitness, sleep and rest, supplementation, cognitive enhancement, and others.

While biohacking has exciting potential, it is critical to weigh the possible benefits against the risks involved. The risks include adverse supplement side effects, over-exertion from exercise, and possible legal issues. As a result, biohackers must proceed with caution, meticulously weighing the risks and benefits of any intervention.

Furthermore, biohacking should not be used in place of conventional medical care, and collaboration with healthcare professionals is required to ensure that interventions are safe and successful. Taking a well-rounded and balanced strategy that integrates multiple strategies and prioritizes safety and sustainability is the key to success.

Overall, biohacking can change the way we think about health and wellness by empowering individuals to take charge of their health and performance. To ensure safe and effective outcomes, it is critical to approach this field with caution and mindfulness, keeping in mind the potential risks and working jointly with healthcare experts.

Key ideas recap

Biohacking is the practice of optimizing and enhancing physical and cognitive function through the use of technology, tools, and lifestyle changes.

Optimizing the body entails improving physical health and efficiency through nutrition, exercise, sleep, and supplementation.

Stress management, meditation, cognitive enhancement, and other methods to improve mental performance are all part of optimizing the mind.

Wearables and tracking devices, biofeedback, cryotherapy, photobiomodulation, and reducing EMF exposure are all examples of biohacking tools and methods.

Biohacking can also be used for anti-aging and longevity tactics like telomere lengthening, caloric restriction, and hormone optimization.

Biohacking can also be used for illness prevention and treatment by optimizing gut health, boosting the immune system, and managing chronic diseases.

Balancing risks and benefits is critical in biohacking because certain methods can have risks and side effects.

Legal issues may also play a role in biohacking, as some methods may be illegal or necessitate medical supervision.

The Biohacking Singularity

The future of biohacking looks promising, as new technologies and innovations appear in the field. Biohacking areas that are expected to see significant growth and development in the coming years include:

CRISPR gene editing technology advances are anticipated to revolutionize the field of biohacking, allowing scientists to make precise edits to the human genome.

Implantable and wearable devices: Wearable technology and implantable devices are expected to become more popular, enabling people to monitor and optimize various aspects of their health in real-time.

Personalized medicine: Biotechnology and data analysis advances are allowing researchers to create personalized treatments and therapies based on an individual's unique genetics, microbiome, and other factors.

Longevity and anti-aging: With new therapies and strategies aimed at extending the human lifespan and increasing health span, the pursuit of anti-aging and longevity is anticipated to remain a major focus of the biohacking community.

Brain-computer interfaces (BCIs): The development of BCIs is likely to usher in a new age of biohacking, allowing people to control machines and even communicate telepathically with one another.

As these and other technologies progress, the field of biohacking is likely to become more mainstream, with more people looking to improve their health and performance through a variety of novel approaches. However, as with any emerging technology, there are risks and ethical considerations to ensure that biohacking is used ethically and for the benefit of society as a whole.

Final ideas and suggestions

Biohacking is a rapidly expanding field that includes the application of science and technology to improve various aspects of human biology and performance. While there are many possible benefits to biohacking, there are also some risks and ethical considerations that should be carefully considered.

To participate in biohacking safely and responsibly, you must:

Begin simple and put safety first: Begin with basic interventions and progress to more advanced methods over time. Before attempting any new intervention, always prioritize safety and confer with a healthcare professional.

Track your progress: Use data tracking tools to track development and determine the effectiveness of interventions.

Concentrate on a comprehensive approach: While biohacking can be used to target specific aspects of health and performance, it is essential to approach it holistically and consider the overall effect.

Keep up with fresh research: Biohacking is a constantly evolving field, and keeping current on new research and advancements is critical for making informed decisions.

Overall, biohacking can change the way we think about health and wellness. We can optimize our biology and reach our maximum potential by combining cutting-edge science and technology with a holistic approach to well-being. However, it is critical to proceed with caution and to always emphasize safety and ethics when it comes to biohacking.